The Ultimate Mediterranean Dinner Guide for Busy People

Super Affordable Recipes to Boost Your Metabolism and Get Back in Shape

Camila Lester

Table of contents

Beet and Caper Salad
Difficulty Level: 2/5

Preparation time: 5 minutes

Cooking time: 25 minutes

Servings: 4

Ingredients

4 medium beets

2 tablespoons of rice wine vinegar

For Dressing

Small bunch parsley, stems removed

1 large garlic clove

½ teaspoon salt

Pinch of black pepper

1 tablespoon extra-virgin olive oil

2 tablespoons capers

Directions:

Pour 1 cup of water into your steamer basket and place it on the side

Snip the tops of your beets and wash them well

Put the beets in your steamer basket

Place the steamer basket in your Pressure Pot and lock the lid

Let it cook for about 25 minutes at high pressure

Once done, release the pressure naturally

While it is being cooked, take a small jar and add chopped up parsley and garlic alongside olive oil, salt, pepper and capers

Shake it vigorously to prepare your dressing

Open the lid once the pressure is released and check the beets for doneness using a fork

Take the steamer basket to your sink and run it under cold water

Use your finger to brush off the skin of the beets

Use a plastic cutting board and slice up the beets

Arrange them on a platter and sprinkle some vinegar on top

Nutrition (Per Serving)

Calories: 231

Fat: 20g

Carbohydrates: 11g

Protein: 2g

Couscous with Tuna and Pepperoncini

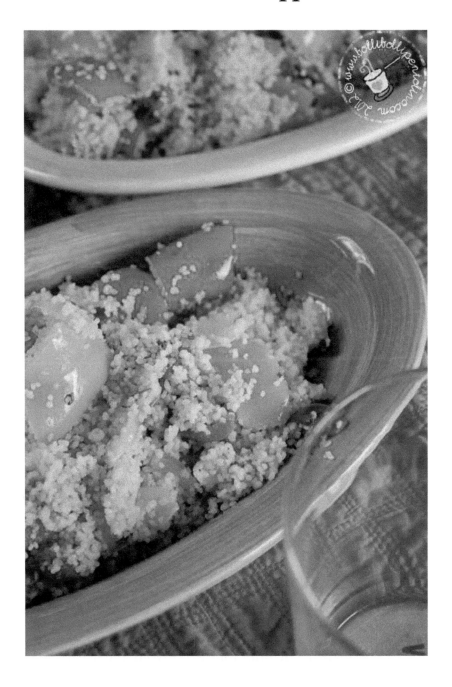

Difficulty Level: 2/5

Preparation time: 10 minutes

Cooking time: 15 minutes

Servings: 4

Ingredients

1 cup chicken broth or water

¾ teaspoon salt

1¼ cups couscous

⅓ cup fresh parsley, chopped

1 lemon, quartered

2 cans (5 oz each) oil packed tuna

1 pint cherry tomatoes, halved

Extra-virgin olive oil (for serving)

½ cup pepperoncini, sliced

¼ cup capers

Salt, pepper, to taste

Directions:

Add 1 cup chicken broth or water to a small pot and boil it. Turn the heat off, stir in 1¼ cups of couscous, and cover it. Let it boil for 10 minutes.

In the meantime, take another bowl and add 1 pint of halved cherry tomatoes, ½ cup of sliced pepperoncini, ¼ cup capers, ⅓ cup fresh chopped parsley, and oil packed tuna; toss well.

Fluff the couscous with a fork. Season with pepper and salt; drizzle with olive oil.

Top with the mixture of tuna and serve your meal with lemon wedges.

Nutritional info (per serving):

226 calories;

10 g fat;

44 g total carbohydrates;

22 g protein

Lemon Chicken with Asparagus
Difficulty Level: 2/5

Preparation time: 10 minutes

Cooking time: 10 minutes

Servings: 3-4

Ingredients

1 lb. boneless skinless chicken breasts

2 tablespoons honey + 2 tablespoons butter

1/4 cup flour

2 lemons, sliced

1/2 teaspoon salt, pepper to taste

1 teaspoon lemon pepper seasoning

1–2 cups asparagus, chopped

2 tablespoons butter

Directions:

Cut the chicken breast in half horizontally. In a shallow dish, mix 1/4 cup flour and salt and pepper to taste; toss the chicken breast until coated.

To a skillet, add 2 tablespoons of butter and melt over medium heat. Then add the coated chicken breast and cook each side for about 4-5 minutes, sprinkling both sides with lemon pepper.

Once chicken is completely cooked through and is golden brown, transfer it to a plate.

For Asparagus and Lemons:

To the pan, add 1–2 cups chopped asparagus; sauté until bright green for a few minutes.

Remove from the pan and keep it aside. Place the slices of lemon to the bottom of the pan and cook each side until caramelized, for a few minutes without stirring.

Add a bit of butter along with the lemon slices. Take the lemons out of the pan and put them aside.

Serve the chicken with the asparagus and enjoy!

Nutritional info (per serving):

232 calories;

9 g fat;

10.4 g total carbs;

27.5 g protein

Cilantro Lime Chicken
Difficulty Level: 2/5

Preparation time: 10 minutes

Cooking time: 12 minutes

Servings: 4

Ingredients

2 tablespoons olive oil

1/4 teaspoon salt

1.5 lb. boneless chicken breast

1/2 teaspoon ground cumin

1/4 cup lime juice

1/4 cup fresh cilantro

For Avocado Salsa*:*

1/2 tablespoon red wine vinegar

Salt, to taste

4 avocados, diced

1 garlic clove, minced

1/2 cup fresh cilantro, diced

1/2 teaspoon red pepper flakes

3 tablespoons lime juice

Directions:

Add cilantro, lime juice, 1/2 teaspoon ground cumin, 2 tablespoons olive oil, and salt to a bowl; whisk well.

Add the marinade and chicken breast to a large Ziploc bag; marinate for about 15 minutes.

Preheat the grill to 400°F. Grill the chicken until it's no longer pink, for about 5-7 minutes per side. Remove from the grill.

For avocado salsa: add lime juice, cilantro, 1/2 tablespoon red wine vinegar, 1/2 teaspoon red pepper flakes, 1 minced clove of garlic, salt, and 4 diced avocados to a blender; process well until smooth.

Serve and enjoy!

Nutritional info (per serving):

317 calories;

22 g fat;

11 g total Carbohydrates;

24 g protein

Shrimp And Leek Spaghetti
Difficulty Level: 2/5

Preparation time: 10 minutes

Cooking time: 20 minutes

Servings: 4

Ingredients:

1 lb. peeled, deveined raw shrimp

8 oz. uncooked whole-grain spaghetti

1 tablespoon garlic, chopped

2 cups leek, chopped

1 ½ tablespoons olive oil

¼ cup heavy cream

2 cups frozen baby sweet peas

2 tablespoons dill, chopped

2 teaspoons lemon zest

2 tablespoons lemon juice

½ teaspoon black pepper

¾ teaspoon kosher salt

Directions:

Cook the pasta according to the package instructions. Drain and reserve ½ cup cooking liquid. Cover the pasta.

Pat dry the shrimp and season with pepper and ¼ teaspoon salt.

Heat half of the oil in a skillet over high heat. Add shrimp and cook for 4 minutes, stirring often. Transfer to a plate and cover.

Reduce the heat to medium high. Add garlic, leek, ½ teaspoon salt, and the remaining oil. Cook for 3 minutes, stirring often.

Add cream, peas, lemon zest, lemon juice, and the reserved liquid. Reduce the heat to medium and cook for 3 minutes. Add the shrimp to the skillet and toss well.

Add the pasta evenly to 4 bowls. Add the sauce and the shrimp on top.

Add dill and serve.

Nutritional info (per serving):

446 calories;

13 g fat;

59 g total carbs;

28 g protein

Lamb and Beet Meatballs

Difficulty Level: 2/5

Preparation time: 5 minutes

Cooking time: 20 minutes

Servings: 4

Ingredients

1 tablespoon olive oil

1 (8 oz.) package beets, cooked

6 oz. ground lamb

1/2 cup bulgur, uncooked

1 teaspoon ground cumin

1/2 cup cucumber, grated

1/2 cup sour cream, reduced-fat

2 tablespoons fresh mint, thinly sliced

2 tablespoons fresh lemon juice

1 oz. almond flour

4 cups mixed baby greens

3/4 teaspoon kosher salt

3/4 teaspoon freshly ground black pepper

Directions:

Preheat the oven to 425F.

Add the beets to a food processor and pulse until finely chopped, Then combine the chopped beets with bulgur, lamb, cumin, ½ teaspoon of salt, pepper, and almond flour in a bowl.

Divide the lamb mixture and shape it into 12 meatballs.

Heat the oil in a skillet over medium-high heat, then add into prepared meatballs. Cook until nicely browned on all sides, for about 4 minutes.

Transfer the browned meatballs to the preheated oven and bake until well cooked, about 8 minutes.

Combine the remaining ¼ teaspoon of salt together with cucumber, juice, mint, and sour cream in a bowl, then divide the greens among the serving plates.

Top the greens with the meatballs evenly and serve with the cucumber mixture. Enjoy!

Nutritional info (per serving):

338 calories;

21 g fat;

25 g total carbs;

14 g protein

Chicken Wings Platter
Difficulty Level: 2/5

Preparation time: 10 minutes

Cooking time: 20 minutes

Servings: 4

Ingredients:

2 pounds chicken wings

½ cup tomato sauce

A pinch of salt and black pepper

1 teaspoon smoked paprika

1 tablespoon cilantro, chopped

1 tablespoon chives, chopped

Directions:

In your Pressure Pot, combine the chicken wings with the sauce and the rest of the ingredients, stir, put the lid on and cook on High for 20 minutes.

Release the pressure naturally for 10 minutes, arrange the chicken wings on a platter and serve as an appetizer.

Nutrition:

Calories 203,

Fat 13g,

Fiber 3g,

Carbohydrates 5g,

Protein 8g

Appetizing Tuna
Difficulty Level: 2/5

Preparation time: 15 min

Cooking time:: - min

Servings: 12

Ingredients:

4 (5 oz.) tuna caned in water, drained

5 hard-boiled eggs, chopped

1/2 cup chopped sweet onion

1 stalk celery, chopped

1 1/2 tablespoons dill pickle relish

2 tsps. honey mustard

3/4 cup mayonnaise

1/2 tsp. celery seed

1/2 tsp. seasoned salt

1/2 tsp. ground black pepper

Directions:

In a large bowl mix together tuna, eggs, onion, and celery.

In a small bowl mix together relish, honey mustard, mayonnaise, celery seed, salt, and pepper.

Combine the mix from the small bowl with the mix from the large bowl, stir gently to coat. Serve at room temperature or let it chill till ready to eat. *Enjoy!*

Nutrition: (Per serving)

Calories:186kcal;

Fat:13.6g;

Saturated fat:2.4g;

Cholesterol:106mg;

Carbohydrate:2g;

Sugar:1g;

Fiber:0.2g;

Protein:13.6g

Avocado and Tuna
Difficulty Level: 2/5

Preparation time: 20 min

Cooking time: - min

Servings: 4

Ingredients:

1 (12 oz.) tuna caned in water, drained

1 tablespoon mayonnaise

3 green onions, thinly sliced, plus, additional for garnish

1 dash balsamic vinegar

black pepper to taste

1 pinch garlic salt, or to taste

2 ripe avocados, halved and pitted

1/2 red bell pepper, chopped

Directions:

In a bowl mix together tuna, red pepper, green onions, and balsamic vinegar. Season with garlic salt and pepper.

With tuna mixture pack the avocado halves. Before serving garnish with green onions and dash of black pepper. *Enjoy!*

Nutrition: (Per serving)

Calories: 294kcal;

Fat: 18.2g;

Saturated fat: 2.8g;

Cholesterol: 27mg;

Carbohydrate: 11g;

Sugar: 1.9g;

Fiber:7.4g;

Protein:23.9g

Grilled Salmon Kebabs One Way

Difficulty Level: 2/5

Preparation time: 10 min

Cooking time: 10 min

Servings: 4

Ingredients:

2 tsp. sesame seeds

2 tbsp. chopped fresh oregano

1/4 tsp. crushed red pepper flakes

1 tsp. ground cumin

2 lemons, very thinly sliced into rounds

extra-virgin (organic) olive oil spray

1 tsp. kosher salt

1 tsp. kosher salt

Directions:

Spray the greats with oil and the grill on medium heat. Combine sesame seeds, oregano, red pepper flakes, and cumin in a small bowl, mix well. Set aside spice mixture.

Onto 8 pairs of parallel skewers treat salmon and folded lemon slices (beginning and ending with salmon), to make 8 kebabs total. Spray the salmon lightly with olive oil and season with salt and reserved spice mixture.

Grill the salmon, turning occasionally, till the salmon is opaque throughout, around 8 – 10 minutes. *Enjoy!*

Nutrition: (Per serving)

Calories:267kcal;

Fat: 11g;

Saturated fat: 2.1g;

Cholesterol: 94mg;

Carbohydrate: 7g;

Sugar: 0g;

Fiber: 3g;

Protein: 35g

Grilled Cedar Plank Salmon
Difficulty Level: 2/5

Preparation time: 10 min

Cooking time: 20 min

Servings: 4

Ingredients:

1 untreated cedar plank

1 (1 1/4 lbs.) boneless wild salmon fillet

1 lemon, halved

1 tsp. dried oregano

3/4 tsp. kosher salt

1/8 tsp. black pepper

few sprigs of fresh oregano and thyme (optional)

1 cup grape tomatoes, halved

1 tsp. extra-virgin olive oil

1 tsp. red wine vinegar

1/4 cup sliced red onion

1/4 cup Kalamata olives, quartered in long strips

1/8 tsp. kosher salt

black pepper, to taste

fresh oregano for garnish

Directions:

Place the cedar plank in water for 1 hour to soak.

Slice into thin slices 1/2 of the lemon. Use the remaining juice from 1/2 of the lemon to season salmon, and also add oregano, salt, and pepper. Cover and refrigerate till ready to grill.

Combine in a medium bowl tomatoes, olive oil, vinegar, red onion, olives, salt, and pepper.

Place on the plank, skin side down, salmon and fresh herbs. Top that whit lemon slices.

Leaving the right burners off (so you have indirect heat) heat the grill to medium-high heat. Close the grill cover and allow the grill to get hot.

Transfer the planked salmon on direct heat side for 3 – 4 minutes, till the plank start to smoke and become a little charred on the bottom and edges (keep a spray bottle with water by your side in case the edges of plank ignite, check occasionally to make sure this don't happen).

After the 3 – 4 minutes have passed, move the planked salmon to the indirect heat side, close the grill cover, and grill for another 12 – 15 minutes based on the thickness, or till the salmon is cooked throughout in the thickest part (use a fork to take a peak)

When the salmon is cooked, cover it with tomato mix and serve. *Enjoy!*

Nutrition: (Per serving)

Calories:251kcal;

Fat:11g;

Saturated fat:1.6g;

Cholesterol:78mg;

Carbohydrate:8g;

Sugar:0g;

Fiber:2g;

Protein:30g

Arugula Salmon Salad

Difficulty Level: 2/5

Preparation time: 10 min

Cooking time: 10 min

Servings: 1

Ingredients:

1 1/2 cups baby arugula

4 oz. sockeye wild salmon, skin removed

1 tsp. capers, drained

2 tsp. red wine vinegar

1 tsp. extra-virgin olive oil

1 tbsp. (.25 oz.) shaved Parmesan cheese

salt and fresh pepper to taste

Directions:

With a little salt and pepper season the wild salmon, and cook for around 10 minutes, either broiled, on the grill, or in a pan lightly sprayed with olive oil. Put arugula on a dish, sprinkle with salt and pepper and cover with salmon and capers. Drizzle vinegar and olive oil on top and finish with fresh shaved Parmesan cheese. *Enjoy!*

Nutrition: (Per serving)

Calories:288kcal;

Fat:16.1g;

Saturated fat:3.1g;

Cholesterol:66.4mg;

Carbohydrate:11g;

Sugar:2g;

Fiber:3g;

Protein:26g

Tilapia With Peppers And Olives
Difficulty Level: 2/5

Preparation time: 10 min

Cooking time: 10 min

Servings: 4

Ingredients:

2 tbsp. extra-virgin olive oil

4 (6-oz.) tilapia fillets

1 onion, thinly sliced

1 onion, thinly sliced

2 red bell peppers, thinly sliced

1/2 cup pitted green olives

1/2 cup fresh flat-leaf parsley, chopped

2 tbsp. fresh lime juice

Directions:

Over medium-high heat in a large non-stick skillet heat 1 tablespoon of olive oil.

With 1/4 teaspoon, each, salt and pepper season the tilapia and cook till opaque throughout, 4 – 5 minutes per side.

In the meantime, over medium-high heat in a second large skillet heat the remaining 1 tablespoon of olive oil.

Stirring often, cook the onion and peppers, till tender, 8 – 10 minutes.

Stir in parsley, olives, lime juice, and 1/4 teaspoon each salt and pepper into the vegetables. Serve with the tilapia. *Enjoy!*

Nutrition: (Per serving)

Calories:276kcal;

Fat:13g;

Saturated fat:3g;

Cholesterol:73mg;

Carbohydrate:8g;

Sugar:3g;

Fiber:3g;

Protein:35g

Cilantro Tilapia
Difficulty Level: 2/5

Preparation time: 5 min

Cooking time: 12 min

Servings: 4

Ingredients:

3 tbsp. extra-virgin olive oil

4 (4 oz.) tilapia fillets, fresh

2 tbsp. garlic salt

2 tbsp. Cajun seasoning

black pepper, to taste

1 bunch cilantro

Directions:

Preheat the oven to 375 degrees Fahrenheit.

Using olive oil coat the bottom of a baking dish.

Arrange tilapia in the pan.

Sprinkle garlic salt, Cajun seasoning, and pepper over tilapia fillets.

Press a few springs of cilantro on top of each tilapia fillet.

Transfer the tilapia into the oven and bake for 8 – 12 minutes. Enjoy alone or with lemon. *Enjoy!*

Tip: Make this into a meal by tossing arugula, baby kale, or other lettuce greens in lemon juice, olive oil, salt and pepper and having as a side salad.

Nutrition: (Per serving)

Calories:200.1kcal;

Fat:12.1g;

Saturated fat:2g;

Cholesterol:56.7mg;

Carbohydrate:0.3g;

Sugar:0.1g;

Fiber:0.2g;

Protein:22.9g

Tilapia Al Ajillo
Difficulty Level: 2/5

Preparation time: 5 min

Cooking time: 15 min

Servings: 4

Ingredients:

1 1/2 lbs. tilapia fillet

4 clove garlic, thinly sliced

3 tbsp. extra-virgin olive oil

salt

pepper

1 lemon, for serving

asparagus

Directions:

Use salt and pepper to season tilapia fillets.

In a skillet heat olive oil over medium heat.

When the olive oil gets hot place tilapia fillets, and when they start to turn color a bit (after 1 – 2 minutes) add garlic slices.

Cook for another 4 minutes or so, then flip the fillets.

Cook the fillets till cooked through, and the fillets flake easily with a fork (this entirely depends on the thickness of your fillets, so keep a close eye on them).

The garlic should get golden brown color, so if you notice that it is starting to burn, spoon it over the fillets, so it is no more in contact with the pan.

When fillets are cooked squeeze freshly lemon juice over them.

Serve with asparagus and garnish with chopped parsley. *Enjoy!*

Nutrition: (Per serving)

Calories:257kcal;

Fat:13g;

Saturated fat:2g;

Cholesterol:85mg;

Carbohydrate:1g;

Sugar:0g;

Fiber:0g;

Protein:34g

Savory Lemon White Fish Fillet

Difficulty Level: 2/5

Preparation time: 15 min

Cooking time: 6 min

Servings: 4

Ingredients:

4 (4 to 6 ounces) cod, halibut, or flounder

6 tablespoons extra-virgin olive oil, divided

1/4 teaspoon kosher or sea salt

1/4 teaspoon freshly ground black pepper

2 lemons, one cut in halves, one cut in wedges

Directions:

For around 10 -15 minutes allow the fish to sit in a bowl at room temperature.

On both side of each fillet rub 1 tablespoon of olive oil and season with salt and pepper.

Over medium heat in a skillet or sauté pan add 2 tablespoons of olive oil. After around 1 minute, when the olive oil is hot and simmering, but not smoking add the fillets. Cook for around 2 – 3 minutes per side, so that each side of fillets are browned and cooked through.

Squeeze lemon halves over the fillets and remove from the heat. Pour over the fillets any lemon juice if left in the pan. Serve with lemon wedges. *Enjoy!*

Tip: Make this into a meal by tossing arugula, baby kale, or other lettuce greens in lemon juice, olive oil, salt and pepper and having as a side salad.

Nutrition: (Per serving)

Calories:197kcal;

Fat:12g;

Saturated fat:2g;

Cholesterol:56mg;

Carbohydrate:1g;

Sugar:0g;

Fiber:0g;

Protein:21g

Shrimp Skewers With Garlic-Lime Marinade

Difficulty Level: 2/5

Preparation time: 15 min

Cooking time: 5 min

Servings:6

Ingredients:

1 pound large raw shrimp, cleaned and deveined

2 tablespoons extra-virgin olive oil

3 cloves garlic, sliced thin

1/4 cup fresh squeezed lime juice

1/4 teaspoon paprika

1/4 teaspoon kosher or sea salt

1/4 teaspoon black pepper

1/4 cup finely chopped cilantro or parsley, for serving

6 large bamboo or metal skewers (if bamboo, soak in warm water 30 minutes prior to cooking)

Directions:

For marinade whisk together olive oil, garlic, lemon juice, paprika, salt, and pepper.

Threat around 5 – 6 shrimps onto each skewer. Place them on the plate and pour marinade over them.

To grill: Set the grill to medium heat and oil the grates with olive oil. Place the skewers to the grill and cook for around 2 minutes per side, or till pink and opaque. Drizzle with any extra marinade while cooking.

To roast in oven: Preheat the oven to 450 degrees Fahrenheit. On the baking sheet place the skewers and roast for around 5 minutes, or till pink and opaque. Garnish with cilantro or parsley before serving, if desired. *Enjoy!*

Nutrition: (Per serving)

Calories:108kcal;

Fat:5g;

Saturated fat:1g;

Cholesterol:122mg;

Carbohydrate:1g;

Sugar:0g;

Fiber:0g;

Protein:15g

Chicken With Olives And Herbs

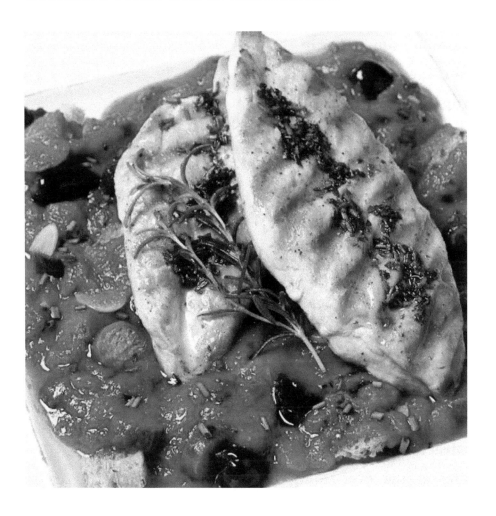

Difficulty Level: 2/5

Preparation time: 10 min

Cooking time: 16 min

Servings: 4

Ingredients:

1/2 tbsp. extra-virgin olive oil

4 (8 oz.) boneless chicken breasts

1/2 tsp kosher salt

2 tsps. all purpose or gluten free flour

1/2 cup dry white wine

1/4 cup lemon juice

2 cloves garlic, crushed

1 tsp. chopped fresh thyme

1 cup pitted chopped olives

1 tbsp. chopped fresh parsley

4 thin lemon slices (optional)

Directions:

Preheat the oven to 400 degrees Fahrenheit with center positioned rack.

Over medium-high heat in a 10-inch cast iron skillet heat the olive oil. Season the chicken with salt and pepper and sprinkle with flour.

Sear chicken when olive oil become hot, sear for around 3 minutes per side.

Add in wine, lemon juice, garlic, thyme, and olives. Top with lemon slices, if desired.

Move the pan to the preheated oven and bake around 10 minutes, until an instant-read thermometer registers 165 degrees Fahrenheit in the center of the thickest part of the chicken.

Serve hot topped with parsley. *Enjoy!*

Nutrition: (Per serving)

Calories:351kcal;

Fat:11g;

Saturated fat:3g;

Cholesterol:166mg;

Carbohydrate:4.5g;

Sugar:0.5g;

Fiber:1g;

Protein:52.5g

Greek Feta-Zucchini Turkey Burgers
Difficulty Level: 2/5

Preparation time: 20 min

Cooking time: 10 min

Servings: 4

Ingredients:

1 lbs. 93% lean ground turkey

1/4 cup seasoned whole wheat breadcrumbs

5 oz. grated zucchini (when squeezed 4 oz.)

2 tbsp. grated red onion

1 clove garlic, crushed

1 tbsp. fresh oregano

3/4 tsp kosher salt and fresh pepper

1/4 cup crumbled feta cheese (from Salad Savors)

extra-virgin (organic) olive oil spray

1 cucumber, diced

3/4 cup quartered grape tomatoes

2 tbsp. chopped red onion

1/3 cup Kalamata olives

1/4 cup roasted peppers

2 tsp. red wine vinegar

1 tsp. fresh oregano

1 tsp. extra-virgin olive oil

kosher salt

1 tbsp. crumbled feta

Ingredients for the salad:

Directions:

Using paper towels squeeze all the moisture from the zucchini.

Combine in a large bowl, mixing well, ground turkey, bread crumbs, zucchini, onion, garlic, oregano, salt, and pepper. Add in 1/4 cup of feta cheese, mix well, and make 5 equally sized patties (not to thick so they can easily be cooked in the center).

Combine in a medium bowl, mixing well, the tomato, cucumber, vinegar, red onion, salt and remaining Feta.

If cooking indoors: Heat, over medium-high heat, large non-stick skillet. Lightly spray olive oil when the skillet is hot. Transfer the burgers to the pan and lower the heat to low. Cook till browned then flip. Flip over a couple of times to prevent the burgers from burning and also to make sure they are cooked all the way through.

If grilling: Before cooking clean the grill and then generously oil the grates to prevent sticking. On medium heat cook the burgers around 5 minutes per side, or till no longer pink in the center.

Transfer the burgers on a dish and top with 2/3 of salad and serve. *Enjoy!*

Nutrition: (Per serving)

Calories:221kcal;

Fat:11g;

Saturated fat:3g;

Cholesterol:73mg;

Carbohydrate:10g;

Sugar:1g;

Fiber:2g;

Protein:20g

Potato Greens Meal

Difficulty Level: 2/5

Preparation time: 10 minutes

Cooking time: 15 minutes

Servings: 4

Ingredients:

4 medium potatoes, cut in large pieces

2 heads of greens (kale, Swiss chard, dandelion, spinach, mustard greens etc.), chopped

1 cup water

Juice of 1 lemon

1 cup extra-virgin olive oil

10 cloves garlic, chopped

Salt and pepper to taste

Directions

Open the top lid of your Pressure Pot.

Add the ingredients; stir to combine with a wooden spatula.

Close the lid and make sure that the valve is sealed properly.

Press MANUAL and set timer to 15 minutes.

The Pressure Pot will start building pressure; allow the mixture to cook for the set time.

When the timer reads zero, press QPR for quick pressure release.

Open the lid and take out the prepared recipe.

Serve warm with some lemon slices.

Nutrition (per serving)

Calories 519,

Fat 13.5 g,

Carbohydrates 34 g,

Protein 4 g,

Sodium 129 mg

Onion Garlic Quinoa
Difficulty Level: 2/5

Preparation time: 10 minutes

Cooking time: 14 minutes

Servings: 6

Ingredients:

1 onion, diced

1 teaspoon minced garlic

2 cups quinoa

1 tablespoon avocado oil or olive oil

2½ cups vegetable broth

Salt and pepper to taste

Directions:

Add the quinoa to a bowl with enough water to submerge. Soak for 1 hour. Drain, wash the quinoa until the water runs clear, and set aside.

Open the top lid of your Pressure Pot and press SAUTÉ.

Add the oil to the pot and heat it.

Add the onions and stir-cook for 7–8 minutes until soft and translucent.

Add the garlic and quinoa; stir-cook for 4–5 minutes until fragrant.

Add the broth, salt and pepper. Stir the mixture.

Close the lid and make sure that the valve is sealed properly.

Press MANUAL and set timer to 1 minute.

The Pressure Pot will start building pressure; allow the mixture to cook for the set time.

When the timer reads zero, press NPR for natural pressure release. It will take 8–10 minutes to release the pressure.

Open the lid and take out the prepared recipe.

Fluff the mixture and serve warm.

Nutrition (per serving)

Calories 242,

Fat 5 g,

Carbs 39 g,

Protein 8 g,

Sodium 395 mg

Lamb Chops with Herb Butter
Difficulty Level: 2/5

Preparation time: 10 minutes

Cooking time: 10 mins

Servings: 4

Ingredients

8 lamb chops

1 tbsp butter

1 tbsp olive oil

Salt

Pepper

4oz herb butter (shop bought)

1 lemon, cut into wedges

Directions:

Season the lamb chops with a little salt and pepper

Add the butter to the pan and wait to melt

Fry the lamb chops in each side for around 4 minutes, depending on thickness

Arrange on a serving plate with a chunk of herb butter and a lemon wedge

Nutrition

Carbs - 0.3g

Fat - 62g

Protein - 43g

Calories - 729

Healthy Lasagna
Difficulty Level: 3/5

Preparation time: 5 minutes

Cooking time: 10 mins

Servings: 4

Ingredients

2 tbsp olive oil

1 onion

1 clove of garlic

20oz beef, ground

3 tbsp tomato paste

0.5 tsp basil, dried

2 tsp salt

0.5 cup of water

0.25 tsp black pepper

8 eggs

10oz cream cheese

5 tbsp psyllium husk powder

2 cups sour cream

5oz cheese, shredded

2oz parmesan cheese, grated

0.5 cup chopped parsley, fresh

Baking tray lined with parchment paper

Large oven proof dish

Directions:

Chop the onion finely, and the garlic

Cook in the olive oil until it has gone soft

Add the ground beef and break up with a spoon as it cooks

Add the garlic, pepper, tomato paste and combine

Add the water and allow to boil, before turning the heat down to a simmer, for around 10 minutes

Meanwhile, you can make the lasagna pasta from scratch - preheat your oven to 150°C

Into a bowl, add the eggs, cream cheese, half the salt and combine well

Add the ground psyllium husk and combine once more, allowing it to rest for a few minutes

Take a baking tray and line with parchment paper

Spread the mixture over the tray in a thin layer, with a second piece of parchment over the top

Place in the oven for 12 minutes

Once cool, remove the paper and slice up the lasagna sheets to pieces which will fit into your oven proof dish

Preheat your oven to 200°C

In a bowl, mix together the sour cream and parmesan, leaving just a little of the parmesan for the topping

Season and add the parsley, combining once more

Take your baking dish and add the lasagna sheets

Add the cheese mixture on top of the sheets

Add the meat sauce on top

Sprinkle some cheese on top and place in the oven

Bake until the cheese has melted

Nutrition

Carbs - 9g

Fat - 76g

Protein - 42g

Calories - 901

Cabbage Stir Fry
Difficulty Level: 2/5

Preparation time: 5 minutes

Cooking time: 5 mins

Servings: 2

Ingredients

5oz butter

20oz ground beef

25oz cabbage (green)

1 tsp salt

1 tsp onion powder

0.25 tsp pepper

1 tbsp white wine vinegar

2 cloves of garlic

3 sliced scallions

1 tsp chilli flakes

1 tbsp chopped ginger, fresh

1 tbsp sesame oil

Directions:

Shred up the cabbage with a food processor

Add the butter to the frying pan and cook the cabbage for a few minutes

Add the vinegar and the spices and combine

Transfer to a bowl

Add the remaining butter to the pan and add the chilli flakes, garlic, and ginger, cooking for a few minutes

Add the meat and wait for the juices to disappear, before turning the heat down a little

Add the cabbage and scallions to the pot and stir well

Season and serve with sesame oil

Nutrition:

Carbs - 10g

Fat - 93g

Protein - 33g

Calories - 1023

Spicy Mexican Casserole

Difficulty Level: 2/5

Preparation time: 5 minutes

Cooking time: 10 mins

Servings: 4

Ingredients

25oz beef, ground

2oz butter

3tbsp Mexican seasoning (Tex Mex works well)

7oz tomatoes, crushed

2oz jalapeños (you can use pickled)

7oz cheese, shredded

1 cup sour cream

1 chopped scallion

5oz iceberg lettuce

Large baking dish, greased

Directions:

Preheat the oven to 200°C

Add the butter to a pan and cook the beef

Add the Mexican seasoning and the tomatoes and cover well

Simmer for 5 minutes and season if necessary

Add the mixture into a baking dish (greased)

Add the peppers and cheese on top

Place in the oven for 20 minutes

In a separate bowl, combine the scallion and sour cream

Remove the casserole and allow to cool a little

Serve with the dip on the side

Nutrition

Carbs - 8g

Fat - 70g

Protein - 50g

Calories - 870

Succulent Baked Salmon
Difficulty Level: 2/5

Preparation time: 5 minutes

Cooking time: 5 mins

Servings: 4

Ingredients

1 tbsp olive oil

2lb salmon

1 tsp salt

7oz butter

1 lemon

A little pepper

Large oven safe dish

Directions:

Preheat your oven to 200°C

Take a large oven safe dish and grease with oil

Arrange the salmon into the dish, with the skin facing upwards

Add salt and pepper

Slice the lemon and butter thinly and place over the top of the salmon

Place into the oven for half an hour

Take the rest of the butter and place into a pan, melting until it bubbles

Stir in a little lemon juice and pour over the salmon

Serve!

Nutrition

Carbs - 1g

Fat - 49g

Protein - 31g

Calories - 573

Coconut Chicken Curry

Difficulty Level: 2/5

Preparation time: 5 minutes

Cooking time: 10 mins

Servings: 4

Ingredients

2 tbsp coconut oil

1 tbsp curry powder

2 lemongrass stalks

20oz boneless chicken thighs

1 small piece of fresh ginger, grated

2 cloves of garlic

1 sliced red bell pepper

14oz coconut cream

0.5 chopped red chilli pepper

Directions:

Cut the lemongrass with a knife, to release the flavour

Cut the chicken up into chunks

Add the coconut oil in a large frying pan and allow to heat up

Cook the ginger, lemongrass and curry powder for a few minutes

Add half of the cut chicken into the pan and cook over a medium temperature

Add salt and pepper and combine

Place the contents of the pan to one side and add the rest of the chicken to the pan

Add the rest of the vegetables to the pan and cook for a few minutes

Add the coconut cream, the other batch of chicken and combine everything together

Allow to simmer for around 10 minutes before serving

Nutrition

Carbs - 8g

Fat - 66g

Protein - 29g

Calories - 736

Blue Cheese Pasta
Difficulty Level: 2/5

Preparation time: 5 minutes

Cooking time: 10 mins

Serves 4

Ingredients

8 eggs

10oz cream cheese

1 tsp salt

5.5 tbsp psyllium husk powder

7oz blue cheese

7oz cream cheese

2oz butter

2 small pinches of black pepper

Baking tray lined with parchment paper

Directions:

Preheat the oven to 150°C

In a bowl, combine the eggs, salt, and cream cheese

Add the psyllium husk a small amount at a time and continue to combine

Allow the bowl to sit to one side for a couple of minutes

Line a baking tray with parchment paper

Spread the batter over the paper and place another piece of parchment over the top

Place in the oven and cook for 12 minutes

Once cooled, remove the paper

Cut into strips with a pizza slicer or a pair of scissors

Take a saucepan and heat over a medium temperature

Add the blue cheese and stir until melted

Add the butter and stir

Pour over the pasta and enjoy

Nutrition

Carbs - 10g

Fat - 87g

Protein 0 37g

Calories - 981

Chicken Alfredo

Difficulty Level: 3/5

Preparation time: 5 minutes

Cooking time: 20 mins

Servings: 4

Ingredients

4 eggs

6 extra egg yolks

2 tbsp olive oil

2.5 tsp salt

30oz chicken breasts, cut into half pieces

10oz bacon, fried

1.25 cup of heavy cream for whipping

0.75 cup of milk, whole

0.75 cup of parmesan cheese

4 cloves of garlic

Pepper

A little butter for cooking

1 cup of water

4 tbsp pesto

6.5 tbsp psyllium husk powder

4 tbsp coconut flour

4 cloves of garlic

8 mushrooms

1 sliced red bell pepper

Baking tray lined with parchment paper

Directions:

Preheat the oven to 150°C

In a separate bowl, mix the eggs, and combine with the olive oil and water

Combine with the psyllium husk powder and coconut flour in a separate bowl

Whisk the dry ingredients into the wet batter and allow to rest for a few minutes

Take a baking tray and line it with parchment paper

Add the batter to the paper and spread out evenly

Place into the oven and cook for 10 minutes

Allow to cool before removing the paper and creating a roll

Cut into strips

Preheat the oven to 200°C

Season the chicken with salt and pepper and cook over a medium heat with the butter

Once cooked, place the chicken into a baking dish and cook for 10 minutes

Meanwhile, fry the bacon

Shred the cheese and add to the bacon, with the cream and milk, bring everything to the boil and stir regularly

Add the garlic and pesto and combine

Add salt and pepper and stir well

Add the mushroom and sliced peppers to a separate frying pan and cook with the butter

Once ready, mix the mushroom sauce and pasta together, tossing well

Serve with the vegetables and the rest of the sauce over the top

Nutrition

Carbs - 12g

Fat - 114g

Protein - 85g

Calories - 1460

Fried Halloumi & Avocados

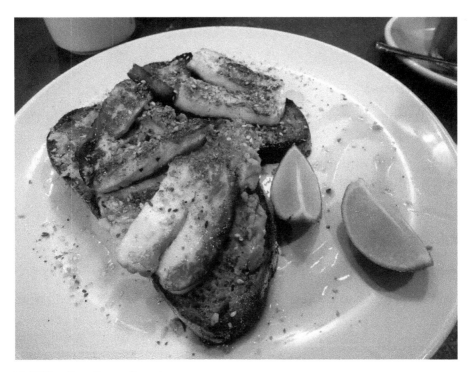

Difficulty Level: 2/5

Preparation time: 5 minutes

Cooking time: 5 mins

Serves 2

Ingredients

10oz halloumi cheese

2 tbsp butter

2 avocados

0.5 cup sour cream

0.25 cucumber

2 tbsp olive oil

2 tbsp pistachio nuts

Salt

Pepper

Directions:

Cut the cheese into slices and add to a frying pan, with the butter for cooking

Cook for a few minutes on each side, until the cheese turns golden and a little gooey

Place the cheese onto a plate

Slice up the cucumber and arrange on the plate

Remove the skin and seed from the avocado and cut into slices

Add the cheese on top of the avocado, drizzle with olive oil and season

Nutrients

Carbs - 12g

Fat - 100g

Protein - 36g

Calories - 1112

Chicken Korma
Difficulty Level: 2/5

Preparation time: 5 minutes

Cooking time: 10 mins

Serves 4

Ingredients

1 sliced red onion

4oz yogurt (Greek yogurt works best)

4 tbsp ghee

3 cloves

1 bay leaf

1 star anise

1 cinnamon stick

3 cardamom pods

8 black peppercorns

15oz chicken thighs, skinless

1 tsp garlic paste

0.5 tsp turmeric

1 tsp red chilli powder

1 tsp coriander seeds, ground

0.5 tsp garam masala

1 tsp cumin, ground

Salt

Directions:

Take a large saucepan and melt the ghee

Once melted, add the onions and cook until they turn golden

Take the onions out and mix in a bowl with the yogurt, blending if necessary

Warm up the ghee once more and add the bay leaf, cloves, star anise, cardamom pods, black peppercorns, and the cinnamon stick

Cook for half a minute

Add the chicken and season with salt

Add the garlic paste and cook for two minutes, stirring often

Add the coriander, garam masala, turmeric, red chilli powder, and cumin, combine well and cook for two more minute

Add the onion and yogurt mixture and combine everything once more

Add a little water and combine

the lid on the pot and cook for 15 minutes

Serve whilst still warm

Nutrition

Carbs - 6g

Fat - 48g

Protein - 27g

Calories - 568

Moroccan Couscous

Difficulty Level: 2/5

Preparation time: 10 minutes

Cooking time: 5 minutes

Servings: 5

Ingredients:

1 cup couscous

1½ cups water

1½ teaspoons grated orange or lemon zest

¾ cup freshly squeezed orange juice

4 or 5 garlic cloves, minced or pressed

2 tablespoons raisins

2 tablespoons pure maple syrup or agave nectar

2¼ teaspoons ground cumin

2¼ teaspoons ground cinnamon

¼ teaspoon paprika

2½ tablespoons minced fresh mint

2 teaspoons freshly squeezed lemon juice

½ teaspoon of sea salt

Directions:

In a medium pot, combine the couscous and water. Add the orange zest and juice, garlic, raisins, maple syrup, cumin, cinnamon, and paprika and stir. Bring the mixture to a boil over medium-high heat.

Remove the couscous from the heat and stir well. Cover with a tight-fitting lid and set aside until all of the liquids are absorbed and the couscous is tender and fluffy. Gently stir in the mint, lemon juice, and salt. Serve warm or cold. Store leftovers in an airtight container in the refrigerator for up to 5 days.

Nutrition:

Calories: 242;

Total Fat: 1g;

Saturated Fat: 0g;

Protein: 7g;

Carbohydrates: 53g;

Fiber: 3g;

Sodium: 244mg;

Iron: 2mg

Alethea's Lemony Asparagus Pasta
Difficulty Level: 2/5

Preparation time: 10 minutes

Cooking time: 20 minutes

Servings: 6

Ingredients:

1 pound spaghetti, linguini, or angel hair pasta

2 crusty bread slices

½ cup plus 1 tablespoon avocado oil, divided

3 cups chopped asparagus (1½-inch pieces)

½ cup vegan "chicken" broth or vegetable broth, divided

6 tablespoons freshly squeezed lemon juice

8 garlic cloves, minced or pressed

3 tablespoons finely chopped fresh curly parsley

1 tablespoon grated lemon zest

1½ teaspoons sea salt

Directions:

Bring a large pot of water to a boil over high heat and cook the pasta until al dente according to the instructions on the package.

Meanwhile, in a medium skillet, crumble the bread into coarse crumbs. Add 1 tablespoon of oil to the pan and stir well to combine over medium heat. Cook for about 5 minutes, stirring often, until the crumbs are golden brown. Remove from the skillet and set aside.

Add the chopped asparagus and ¼ cup of broth in the skillet and cook over medium-high heat until the asparagus is bright green and crisp-tender, about 5 minutes. Transfer the asparagus to a very large bowl.

73

Add the remaining ½ cup of oil, remaining ¼ cup of broth, lemon juice, garlic, parsley, zest, and salt to the asparagus bowl and stir well.

When the noodles are done, drain well, and add them to the bowl. Gently toss with the asparagus mixture. Just before serving, stir in the toasted bread crumbs. Store leftovers in an airtight container in the refrigerator for up 2 days.

Nutrition:

Calories: 526;

Total Fat: 23g;

Saturated Fat: 3g;

Protein: 13g;

Carbohydrates: 68g;

Fiber: 10g;

Sodium: 1422mg;

Iron: 6mg

Mediterranean Grilled Shrimp

Difficulty Level: 2/5

Preparation time: 20 minutes

Cooking time: 5 minutes

Servings: 4-7

Ingredients:

2 tablespoons garlic, minced

½ cup lemon juice

3 tablespoons fresh Italian parsley, finely chopped

¼ cup extra-virgin olive oil

1 teaspoon salt

2 pounds jumbo shrimp (21-25), peeled and deveined

Directions:

In a large bowl, mix the garlic, lemon juice, parsley, olive oil, and salt.

Add the shrimp to the bowl and toss to make sure all the pieces are coated with the marinade. Let the shrimp sit for 15 minutes.

Preheat a grill, grill pan, or lightly oiled skillet to high heat. While heating, thread about 5 to 6 pieces of shrimp onto each skewer.

Place the skewers on the grill, grill pan, or skillet and cook for 2 to 3 minutes on each side until cooked through. Serve warm.

Nutrition:

Calories: 402;

Protein: 57g;

Total Carbohydrates: 4g;

Sugars: 1g;

Fiber: 0g;

Total Fat: 18g;

Italian Breaded Shrimp
Difficulty Level: 2/5

Preparation time: 10 minutes

Cooking time: 5 minutes

Servings: 4

Ingredients:

2 large eggs

2 cups seasoned Italian breadcrumbs

1 teaspoon salt

1 cup flour

1 pound large shrimp (21-25), peeled and deveined

Extra-virgin olive oil

Directions:

In a small bowl, beat the eggs with 1 tablespoon water, then transfer to a shallow dish.

Add the breadcrumbs and salt to a separate shallow dish; mix well.

Place the flour into a third shallow dish.

Coat the shrimp in the flour, then egg, and finally the breadcrumbs. Place on a plate and repeat with all of the shrimp.

Preheat a skillet over high heat. Pour in enough olive oil to coat the bottom of the skillet. Cook the shrimp in the hot skillet for 2 to 3 minutes on each side. Take the shrimp out and drain on a paper towel. Serve warm.

Nutrition:

Calories: 714;

Protein: 37g;

Total Carbohydrates: 63g;

Sugars: 4g;

Fiber: 3g;

Total Fat: 34g

Fried Fresh Sardines

Preparation time: 5 minutes

Cooking time: 5 minutes

Servings: 4

Ingredients:

Avocado oil

1½ pounds whole fresh sardines, scales removed

1 teaspoon salt

1 teaspoon freshly ground black pepper

2 cups flour

Directions:

Preheat a deep skillet over medium heat. Pour in enough oil so there is about 1 inch of it in the pan.

Season the fish with the salt and pepper.

Dredge the fish in the flour so it is completely covered.

Slowly drop in 1 fish at a time, making sure not to overcrowd the pan.

Cook for about 3 minutes on each side or just until the fish is golden brown on all sides. Serve warm.

Nutrition:

Calories: 794;

Protein: 48g;

Total Carbohydrates: 44g;

Fiber: 2g;

Total Fat: 47g

White Wine–Sautéed Mussels

Difficulty Level: 2/5

Preparation time: 10 minutes

Cooking time: 10 minutes

Servings: 4

Ingredients:

3 pounds live mussels, cleaned

4 tablespoons (½ stick) salted butter

2 shallots, finely chopped

2 tablespoons garlic, minced

2 cups dry white wine

Directions:

Scrub the mussel shells to make sure they are clean; trim off any that have a beard (hanging string). Put the mussels in a large bowl of water, discarding any that are not tightly closed.

In a large pot over medium heat, cook the butter, shallots, and garlic for 2 minutes.

Add the wine to the pot, and cook for 1 minute.

Add the mussels to the pot, toss with the sauce, and cover with a lid. Let cook for 7 minutes. Discard any mussels that have not opened.

Serve in bowls with the wine broth.

Nutrition:

Calories: 777;

Protein: 82g;

Total Carbohydrates: 29g;

Sugars: 1g;

Total Fat: 27g;

Saturated Fat: 10g

Chicken Shawarma
Difficulty Level: 2/5

Preparation time: 15 minutes

Cooking time: 15 minutes

Servings: 4

Ingredients:

2 pounds boneless and skinless chicken

½ cup lemon juice

½ cup extra-virgin olive oil

3 tablespoons minced garlic

1½ teaspoons salt

½ teaspoon freshly ground black pepper

½ teaspoon ground cardamom

½ teaspoon cinnamon

Hummus and pita bread, for serving (optional)

Directions:

Cut the chicken into ¼-inch strips and put them into a large bowl.

In a separate bowl, whisk together the lemon juice, olive oil, garlic, salt, pepper, cardamom, and cinnamon.

Pour the dressing over the chicken and stir to coat all of the chicken.

Let the chicken sit for about 10 minutes.

Heat a large pan over medium-high heat and cook the chicken pieces for 12 minutes, using tongs to turn the chicken over every few minutes.

Serve with hummus and pita bread, if desired.

Nutrition:

Calories: 477;

Protein: 47g;

Total Carbohydrates: 5g;

Sugars: 1g;

Fiber: 1g;

Total Fat: 32g

Paprika-Spiced Fish
Difficulty Level: 2/5

Preparation time: 5 minutes

Cooking time: 10 minutes

Servings: 4

Ingredients:

4 (5-ounce) sea bass fillets

½ teaspoon salt

1 tablespoon smoked paprika

3 tablespoons unsalted butter

Lemon wedges

Directions:

Season the fish on both sides with the salt. Repeat with the paprika.

Preheat a skillet over high heat. Melt the butter.

Once the butter is melted, add the fish and cook for 4 minutes on each side.

Once the fish is done, move to a serving dish and squeeze lemon over the top.

Nutrition:

Calories: 257;

Protein: 34;

Total Carbohydrates: 1g;

Fiber: 1g;

Total Fat: 13g

Greek Style Spring Soup
Difficulty Level: 2/5

Preparation Time: 10 minutes

Cooking time: 20 minutes

Servings: 4

Ingredients:

3 cups chicken stock

½ pound chicken breast, shredded

1 tablespoon chives, chopped

1 egg, whisked

½ white onion, diced

1 bell pepper, chopped

1 tablespoon olive oil

¼ cup Arborio rice

½ teaspoon salt

1 tablespoon fresh cilantro, chopped

Directions:

Pour olive oil in the stock pan and preheat it.

Add onion and bell pepper. Roast the vegetables for 3-4 minutes. Stir them from time to time.

After this, add rice and stir well.

Cook the ingredients for 3 minutes over the medium heat.

Then add chicken stock and stir the soup well.

Add salt and bring the soup to boil.

Add shredded chicken breast, cilantro, and chives. Add egg and stir it carefully.

Close the lid and simmer the soup for 5 minutes over the medium heat.

Remove the cooked soup from the heat.

Nutrition:

Calories 176

Fat 5.6 g

Fiber 7.6g

Carbohydrates 23.6 g

Protein 4.6 g

Avgolemono Soup
Difficulty Level: 2/5

Preparation Time: 10 minutes

Cooking time: 20 minutes

Servings: 6

Ingredients:

4 cups chicken stock

1 cup of water

1-pound chicken breast, shredded

1 cup of rice, cooked

3 egg yolks

3 tablespoons lemon juice

1/3 cup fresh parsley, chopped

½ teaspoon salt

¼ teaspoon ground black pepper

Directions:

Pour water and chicken stock in the saucepan and bring to boil.

Then pour one cup of the hot liquid in the food processor.

Add cooked rice, egg yolks, lemon juice, and salt. Blend the mixture until smooth.

After this, transfer the smooth rice mixture into the saucepan with remaining chicken stock liquid.

Add shredded chicken breast, parsley, and ground black pepper.

Boil the soup for 5 minutes more.

Nutrition:

Calories 235

Fat 5.6 g

Fiber 7.6g

Carbohydrates 23.6 g

Protein 4.6 g

Rosemary Minestrone
Difficulty Level: 2/5

Preparation Time: 5 minutes

Cooking time: 25 minutes

Servings: 4

Ingredients:

2 oz celery stalk, chopped

1 russet potato, chopped

½ cup butternut squash, chopped

1 teaspoon fresh rosemary

½ teaspoon salt

½ teaspoon ground black pepper

2 oz Parmesan, grated

1 tablespoon butter

½ zucchini, chopped

¼ cup green beans, chopped

2 oz whole wheat pasta

4 cups chicken stock

½ teaspoon tomato paste

¾ cup red kidney beans, canned, drained

Directions:

In the saucepan combine together celery stalk, potato, butternut squash, rosemary, salt, ground black pepper, butter, and stir well.

Cook the vegetables for 5 minutes over the medium-low heat.

After this, add zucchini, green beans, whole-wheat pasta, chicken stock, and tomato paste.

Add red kidney beans and chicken stock.

Stir the soup well and cook it for 15 minutes over the medium-high heat.

Then add Parmesan and stir minestrone.

Cook it for 2 minutes more.

Ladle minestrone in the serving bowls immediately.

Nutrition:

Calories 234

Fat 6.5

Fiber 10.1

Carbohydrates 39.7

Protein 31.1

Orzo Soup with Kale

Difficulty Level: 2/5

Preparation Time: 10 minutes

Cooking time: 20 minutes

Servings: 4

Ingredients:

1/3 cup orzo pasta

¼ white onion, diced

1 oz celery stalk, chopped

½ teaspoon chili flakes

½ teaspoon salt

1 garlic clove, diced

1 cup kale, chopped

½ cup tomatoes, chopped

1 carrot, chopped

½ teaspoon dried thyme

½ teaspoon dried oregano

5 cups vegetable stock

Directions:

Pour the vegetable stock in the pan and bring it to boil.

Add celery stalk and diced onion.

After this, sprinkle the liquid with chili flakes and salt.

Add diced garlic, tomatoes, carrot, dried thyme, and dried oregano.

Bring the liquid to boil.

Add orzo pasta and cook it for 5 minutes.

After this, add kale and cook the soup for 3 minutes more.

Remove the soup from the heat and leave it to rest with the closed lid for 10 minutes.

Nutrition:

Calories 74

Fat 6.5

Fiber 5.1

Carbohydrates 2.7

Protein 3.1

Braised Swiss Chard with Potatoes
Difficulty Level: 2/5

Preparation time: 5 minutes

Cooking time: 5 minutes

Serving: 4

Ingredients:

1 pound Swiss chard, torn, chopped with stems

2 potatoes, peeled and chopped

¼ tablespoon oregano

1 teaspoon salt

Directions:

Take a pot and add Swiss chard and potatoes to the pot

Pour water to cover all and sprinkle with salt

Close the lid and then press the Pressure cook/Manual button

Cook for 3 minutes on High

Release the steam naturally over 5 minutes

Sprinkle with Italian seasoning or oregano on top

Serve and enjoy!

Nutrition: (Per Serving)

Calories: 246

Fat: 10g

Carbohydrates: 29g

Protein: 12g

Mushroom and Vegetable Penne Pasta
Difficulty Level: 2/5

Preparation Time: 5 minutes

Cooking Time: 8 minutes

Serving: 4

Ingredients:

6 ounces penne pasta

6 ounces shitake mushrooms, chopped

1 small carrot, cut into strips

4 ounces baby spinach, finely chopped

1 teaspoon ginger, grounded

3 tablespoons oil

2 tablespoons soy sauce

6 ounces zucchini, cut into strips

6 ounces leek, finely chopped

½ teaspoon salt

2 garlic cloves, crushed

2 cups of water

Directions:

Heat the oil

Sauté and stir-fry carrot and garlic for 3-4 minutes

Add remaining ingredients and pour in 2 cups water

Cook on High pressure for 4 minutes

Quick-release the pressure

Serve and enjoy!

Nutrition: (Per Serving)

Calories: 429

Fat: 8g

Carbohydrates: 64g

Protein: 25g

Mushroom Spinach Tagliatelle

Difficulty Level: 2/5

Preparation time: 10 minutes

Cooking time: 5 minutes

Serving: 4

Ingredients:

1 pound tagliatelle

¼ cup parmesan cheese, grated

2 garlic cloves, crushed

¼ cup heavy cream

6 ounces mixed mushrooms, frozen

3 tablespoons coconut oil, unsalted

¼ cup feta cheese

1 tablespoon Italian seasoning mix

Directions:

Melt coconut oil on sauté

Stir-fry the garlic for a minute

Stir in feta and mushrooms

Add tagliatelle and 2 cups of water

Cook for 4 minutes on High pressure

Quick-release the pressure

Top with the parmesan

Serve and enjoy!

Nutrition: (Per Serving)

Calories: 298

Fat: 13g

Carbohydrates: 28g

Protein: 14g

Broccoli and Orecchiette Pasta with Feta

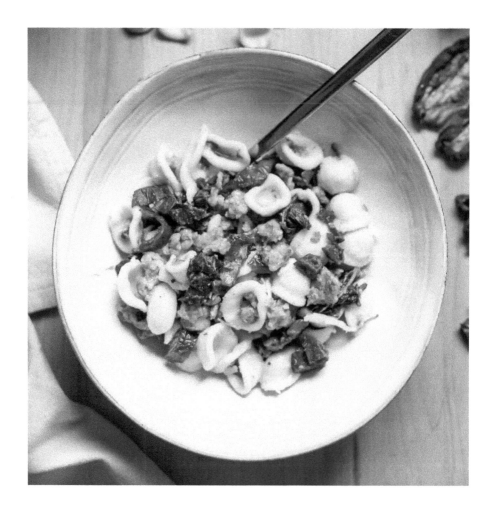

Difficulty Level: 2/5

Preparation time: 10 minutes

Cooking time: 14 minutes

Serving: 4

Ingredients:

1 pack (9 ounces) orecchiette

1 tablespoon feta, grated

16 ounces broccoli, roughly chopped

2 garlic cloves

1 teaspoon salt

¼ teaspoon black pepper

3 tablespoons olive oil

Directions:

Add broccoli and orecchiette into your Pressure Pot

Cover with water and close the lid

Cook on High pressure for 10 minutes

Quick-release the pressure

Drain the broccoli and orecchiette

Set them aside and then heat the oil on sauté mode

Stir-fry garlic for 2 minutes

Stir in orecchiette, broccoli, salt and pepper

Cook for 2 minutes more

Once cooked, then press cancel and stir in grated feta

Serve and enjoy!

Nutrition: (Per Serving)

Calories: 350

Fat: 20g

Carbohydrates: 32g

Protein: 15g

Lentil Spread with Parmesan
Difficulty Level: 2/5

Preparation time: 10 minutes

Cooking time: 7 minutes

Servings: 6

Ingredients:

1 pound lentils, cooked

½ teaspoon oregano, ground

2 tablespoons Parmesan cheese

1 cup sweet corn

2 tomatoes, diced

3 tablespoons tomato paste

1 teaspoon salt

½ teaspoon red pepper flakes

¼ cup red wine

1 cup of water

3 tablespoons olive oil

Directions:

Heat oil on sauté

Add tomatoes, tomato paste, ½ cup water

Sprinkle with salt and oregano and stir-fry for 5 minutes

Press cancel and add sweet corn, wine, and lentils

Pour the remaining water and close the lid

Cook on High pressure for 2 minutes

Quick-release the pressure and set aside for 30 minutes

Add Parmesan cheese on top

Serve and enjoy!

Nutrition (Per Serving)

Calories: 356

Fat: 6g

Carbohydrates: 60g

Protein: 19g

Cod on Millet
Difficulty Level: 2/5

Preparation time: 10 minutes

Cooking time: 7 minutes

Serving: 4

Ingredients:

4 cod fillets

1 yellow bell pepper, diced

1 red bell pepper, diced

2 cups chicken broth

1 tablespoon olive oil

1 cup millet

1 cup breadcrumbs

4 tablespoons coconut oil, melted

¼ cup fresh cilantro, minced

1 teaspoon salt

Directions:

Take a pot and combine the millet, red and yellow bell pepper and oil

Cook for 1 minute on Sauté

Then mix the chicken broth

Place a trivet on top

Take a bowl and mix coconut oil, cilantro, lemon zest, crumbs, juice and salt

Spread the breadcrumb mixture evenly on the cod fillet

Place the fish on the trivet, then close the lid

Cook for 6 minutes on High

Quick release the pressure

Serve and enjoy!

Nutrition (Per Serving)

Calories: 352

Fat: 19g

Carbohydrates: 31g

Protein: 14g

Steamed Sea Bass with Turnips
Difficulty Level: 2/5

Preparation time: 10 minutes

Cooking time: 8 minutes

Ingredients:

4 sea bass fillets

4 sprigs thyme

1 white onion, cut into thin rings

2 turnips, chopped

1½ cups of water

1 lemon, sliced

2 pinches salt

1 pinch ground black pepper

2 teaspoons olive oil

Directions:

Add water and set a rack into the pot

Line a parchment paper at the bottom of the steamer basket

Place the lemon slices in a single layer on the rack

Arrange fillets on the top of the lemons, cover with onion and thyme sprigs, then top with turnip

Add olive oil, salt, and pepper to the mixture

Put the steamer basket onto the rack

Close the lid and cook for 8 minutes on low pressure

Quick-release the pressure

Serve over the onion rings and turnips

Enjoy!

Nutrition (Per Serving)

Calories: 226

Fat: 9g

Carbohydrates: 12g

Protein: 26g

Baked Potato and BBQ Lentils

Difficulty Level: 2/5

Preparation time: 5 minutes

Cooking time: 20 minutes

Servings: 4

Ingredients:

2 large-sized potatoes, baked, cut up into 6 wedges

3 cups of water

2 teaspoons molasses

2 teaspoons liquid smoke

1 cup dry brown lentils

1 small onion, chopped up

½ cup organic ketchup

Directions:

Add water, onion, and lentils to the pot

Close the lid and cook on HIGH pressure for 10 minutes

Release the pressure naturally

Add liquid smoke molasses and ketchup to the lentil

Sauté for 5 minutes

Serve over baked potatoes

Enjoy!

Nutrition (Per Serving)

Calories: 140

Fat: 4g

Carbohydrates: 24g

Protein: 5g

Hearty Lamb Bean

Difficulty Level: 2/5

Preparation time: 5 minutes

Cooking time: 25 minutes

Servings: 6

Ingredients:

28 ounces diced tomato, canned

2 cups beef broth

1½ cup mixed beans, soaked for 12 hours and drained

1½ pounds lamb, ground

1 tablespoon paprika

Salt and pepper, to taste

Directions:

Add all ingredients into your Pressure Pot

Stir gently

Close the pot

Cook for 25 minutes on High pressure on the Stew/Meat setting

Release the pressure naturally

Serve and enjoy!

Nutrition (Per Serving)

Calories: 427

Fat: 12.6g

Carbohydrates: 19.4g

Protein: 27.6g

Mediterranean Kale Dish

Difficulty Level: 2/5

Preparation time: 15 minutes

Cooking time: 10 minutes

Ingredients:

12 cups kale, chopped

2 tablespoons lemon juice

1 teaspoon soy sauce

1 tablespoon olive oil

Salt and pepper, as needed

Directions:

Add a steamer insert to your saucepan

Add water and fill it up to the bottom

Cover and bring water to boil on medium-high heat

Add kale into the insert and steam for 7-8 minutes

Add lemon juice, olive oil, soy sauce, salt and pepper in a large bowl

Mix them well

Add the steamed kale to bowl, toss them

Serve and enjoy!

Nutrition (Per Serving)

Calories: 30

Fat: 17g

Carbohydrates: 41g

Protein: 4g

Greek Orzo Salad

Difficulty Level: 2/5

Preparation time: 5 minutes

Cooking time: 10 minutes

Servings: 4

Ingredients:

1 cup orzo pasta, uncooked

6 tablespoons olive oil

1 onion, chopped

½ cup parsley, minced

1 onion, chopped

1½ teaspoons oregano

Directions:

Cook your orzo and drain them

Add to a serving dish

Add 2 teaspoons oil

Take another dish and add onion, remaining oil, oregano, parsley

Then season with salt and pepper

Pour the mixture over the orzo

Let it chill for 24 hours

Serve and enjoy!

Nutrition (Per Serving)

Calories: 327

Fat: 18g

Carbohydrates: 32g

Protein: 10g

Asparagus Salad
Difficulty Level: 2/5

Preparation time: 10 minutes

Cooking time: 20 minutes

Servings: 4

Ingredients:

1 lemon, juiced

2 salmon fillets

1 tablespoon red wine vinegar

1 tablespoon walnut oil

1 tablespoon Dijon mustard

¼ cup goat Parmesan cheese, shredded

¼ cup fresh mint

¼ cup pine nuts, roasted

¼ teaspoon pepper

2 cups asparagus, shaved

Directions:

Season salmon with salt and keep it on the side

Place a trivet in your Pot

Place salmon over the trivet and close lid, cook on HIGH pressure for 15 minutes

Quick-release pressure

Transfer salmon to a platter and keep it on the side

Add asparagus around the salmon

Take a small bowl and mix lemon juice, walnut oil, champagne vinegar, mustard, and whisk well

Drizzle the dressing over salmon and asparagus

Garnish with pine nuts, pepper, mint and cheddar cheese

Serve and enjoy!

Nutrition (Per Serving)

Calories: 166

Fat: 14g

Carbohydrates: 6g

Protein: 3g

Lightning Source UK Ltd.
Milton Keynes UK
UKHW020745030621
384855UK00001B/190

9 781802 697384